As She Was Dying

As She Was Dying

✦

An Alzheimer's Journal

Mary Wilhoit

iUniverse, Inc.
New York Lincoln Shanghai

As She Was Dying
An Alzheimer's Journal

iUniverse books may be ordered through booksellers or by contacting:

iUniverse
2021 Pine Lake Road, Suite 100
Lincoln, NE 68512
www.iuniverse.com
1-800-Authors (1-800-288-4677)

Because of the dynamic nature of the Internet, any Web addresses or links contained in this book may have changed since publication and may no longer be valid.

The information, ideas, and suggestions in this book are not intended as a substitute for professional medical advice. Before following any suggestions contained in this book, you should consult your personal physician. Neither the author nor the publisher shall be liable or responsible for any loss or damage allegedly arising as a consequence of your use or application of any information or suggestions in this book.

ISBN: 978-0-595-48139-2 (pbk)
ISBN: 978-0-595-60234-6 (ebk)

Printed in the United States of America

Contents

INTRODUCTION: Where We Were ix

OLD FOLKS 1

CONSIDER HER WAYS 3

WATERLINES 4

SOURPUSS 5

MY LITTLE RUNAWAY 7

DRUG FREE MISERY 8

REMEMBERING 9

SELF-EVALUATION 12

GODIVA 13

GOOD DRUGS 14

ZOLOFT SPELLS HOPE? 16

AUTUMN IN THE AIR 18

FURTHER EXPLORATION 19

TRIVIA 22

TRIVIA, TOO 24

SMALL REVELATION 25

INJURY 26

DOWN-TIME 27

TERMS OF ENDEARMENT I 29

TERMS OF ENDEARMENT II 30

TURN-OVER. 31

PREP TIME 33

PONDERING 34

DEPRESSION 36

ON THE ROAD AGAIN. 38

WHEELCHAIRS 39

NEW STAGE. 40

FLASH 42

TODAY 43

POST-OP 44

CHRISTMAS DAY. 45

NEW YEAR'S DAY 47

THE BEAT GOES ON 48

STATUS. 49

PUREE 50

WEDNESDAY 51

GOODBYES. 53

CATCH-UP 54

SUNDAY 55

MONDAY 56

TUESDAY 57

THURSDAY. 58

CONCLUSION: Here and Now 59

THANKS I 61

THANKS II 63

THANKS III 65

THANKS IV 67

FUNEREAL MATTERS 69

LIFE BEGINS ANEW 73

EVALUATION 75

TIME'S WINGED CHARIOT 77

INTRODUCTION:
Where We Were

When we moved my mother from Mississippi to Alabama in the spring of 1993, we didn't realize that she had Alzheimer's. We thought she was merely having problems remembering things. She had always been so independent in so many ways that we never thought to question behavior that we should have viewed as eccentric, to say the least.

In the fall of 1993, I took her to several doctors who performed tests: an upper G.I., a lower endoscopy, and a few other assorted tests. It was clear by then that she had developed dementia, but no one had labeled the cause of her dementia at that time. They just smiled and sent us home. It was quite a while later before someone—and I forget who it was now—finally confirmed what had slowly become clear. My mother had Alzheimer's.

What follows is by no means a thorough account of what happened between the Fall of 1992, when she became very ill with near-pneumonia, attracting our attention to the necessity of dealing with the matter of her health, and the earlier months of 1997. For the portion of that period when she didn't need constant supervision, she lived in a three bedroom house, purchased for her here in Montevallo. During that time, I lived in an adjacent house on the same property. I was an overseer, preparing her meals, arranging for housecleaning services, and, eventually, providing many other services.

In August, 1995, she suffered some kind of stroke-like spell that necessitated hospitalization. When she was released, it was with a seemingly diminished capacity to walk. However, she was given a walker, and, rapidly, because of diligent practice, she regained her walking skills. Still, it was obvious that I needed to move into her house and live with her because she needed more supervision and care than she had before.

Perhaps, I was just tired. I don't know. However, by the end of September, 1995, I was experiencing suicidal thoughts, and my younger son said that I needed to get out. With great relief and gratitude, I moved out of my mother's house into another, while my son moved into her house. His girl friend, who is a registered nurse, moved into the house where I had previously lived alongside my mother. This situation continued, with the introduction of the use of daycare facilities, from late 1995 through the autumn of 1996.

Beginning in the summer of 1996, I began to pick up my mother at daycare in the afternoons and bring her home. By the end of the summer, my son appeared to me to be beginning to feel the need of some weekend relief time, which was quite understandable. He tried hiring a local woman to stay over the weekends, but that didn't work out. Therefore, I volunteered to sit on weekends, inasmuch as I was feeling much better by then.

After a while my son and I discussed the situation, and we decided that a sensible arrangement would be to alternate months keeping my mother in our houses. When I kept her, I would both take her to and retrieve her from daycare and would keep her on weekends. It was at this point that I began to keep a journal on the message boards of America Online, recording some of the events and my feelings about the period. That journal, with some editing and a few additions, is what follows. It was my original intent to give myself an outlet for expression of the varied emotions I was feeling, and, maybe, to offer something with which other people in similar situations could empathize, so that we might all know we were not entirely alone. Judging from reactions, I would say that it served its intended purpose.

OLD FOLKS

Wed, 2 October 96

After spending nearly a year with my younger son, my mother is living with me again. She is 83 now, a former schoolteacher, with a B.A. in English, an M.Ed. in Business Education, equivalent Master's hours in English, a teacher's license, and with credits accumulated towards a Master's in Library Science. She really enjoyed going to school, and she seemed to like teaching school and coaching girls' basketball teams, which she did for at least 30 years. Her high school girls' team at Camp Ground High School in Yalobusha County, Mississippi, won the state championship one year, back in the thirties.

She grew up on a farm in the country in northwest Mississippi, chopping and hoeing endless rows of corn and cotton after her father died as the result of an accident with a firearm that proved to be loaded. Consequently, she developed a strong and healthy body. Even now, in the last days of her life, she still has remarkable strength.

When she finally decided back in late 1992, after becoming very ill, to let me liquidate the family property in Mississippi and move her over here to Alabama, she had great plans for what she was going to do here in this small southern college town. Studying in the library. Attending cultural events. It sounded good, but, unfortunately, she was already much further gone into Alzheimer's than I had realized, and much too far gone to be able to carry out the agenda she seemed to have fashioned. I had just thought that she was being peculiar, and, truth to tell, I think she had always been a few slices short of a loaf. She had functioned—energetically, enthusiastically, obsessively, and oddly.

And so here we are now. When it became clear last year that she was going to need a great deal more tending than she had in the past, we began considering the options. I was told that if we applied for Medicaid, the government would demand all assets that might be traced and/or connected to her for the past three years. Now I'm told that it can be taken back farther still. In other words, the government wants to make sure it gets its hands on as much of what was in her name as it can. The trouble is, the move was expensive in a number of ways.

Those assets can't simply be handed over upon request. If we put her full-time in a nursing home, I—who had taken early retirement to look after her—will have to go back to work, and it would take most of what I might make to keep her in a home. The benefits she receives were quite adequate at the time of my father's death in 1986, but they fall short now. A good home here in Alabama will cost in excess of $3000 per month. So, in the meantime, we send her to daycare during the week. At night and on the weekends, however, she requires a fair amount of supervision. Especially on the weekends.

She wakes very early. This morning when I went to get her, I discovered that she had taken all the linens off the bed and stacked them in various places around the room. That's okay. What I dread—and they will come—are the mornings when I will discover that she has stowed feces around her room. That's what she has been doing at my son's house. He would go into the kitchen in the morning and discover feces on the kitchen counter and, possibly, in the silverware drawer. We have managed to deal with the feces-in-the-kitchen problem, but what she does in her room is another matter.

Perhaps when families were less insular, it was easier to deal with our elderly, but having aging relatives with Alzheimer's nowadays is a wholly new problem. These relatives can occupy all of your life if you are not careful. Caring for them becomes what your life is about.

Perhaps when it is a matter of tending a much-loved parent, it makes a difference. I have a feeling, however, that there comes a point when, much-loved or not, we caregivers begin to break under the pressure. I've had most of the last year off, but it's my turn again.

With the growing mass of the aged, lots of us are going to have a turn in the near future. If this is a potential problem for you, you need to start giving the matter a little thought, so that when the time comes, you will be ready. I wish I had.

CONSIDER HER WAYS

Fri, 4 October 96

Well, we learn something every day. I learned last night that putting my mom in pajamas that button down the front is not the way to go. This was a pair of flannels that she has worn a lot and that she recently stained with fecal matter. I have washed them thoroughly, but they are still stained, and, I imagine, will remain so. The mom has been wearing sweats to daycare all summer because she stays fairly cold. With her eating habits she just isn't very fleshy anymore.

Anyway, after we had gotten the pajamas on and buttoned, she became concerned that there wasn't a button near the bottom edge of the jacket front. This we solved with the use of a safety pin. So far, so good. Then, however, she began to want to button the jacket up to the neck. The object there that looked like a fastener, if it actually ever was one, has not operated in ages. I'm afraid I had lost my patience by then. She sat (after a lot of convincing) for maybe 30 minutes, obsessing about the neck closure, fumbling and fingering it and wrapping the pajamas around her tightly.

Lesson learned? From now on, it's sweats for the night. Night and day. It is the only way she can begin to stay warm, and they have no buttons.

WATERLINES

Sat, 22 February 97

This is an anecdote, remembered and written about in another folder on-line:

During the 93–94 school year the mom was in such a state that she could be left in her house by herself, or at least I thought so. At any rate, I couldn't stand living with her, so it had to work. I was living in a smaller house on the same property, about 30 ft. further back and across a driveway. One warmish winter day, my mother said she had something she wanted to show me—to ask about. So I let her lead me to the front of my house where, alongside a water faucet that jutted out from the base of the house, there was a ladder leaning against the wall. Draped across and over a rung of the ladder, about waist high, was a garden hose without a nozzle. My mother directed my attention to the mouth of the hose. Some drops of water were falling from it to the ground.

"It's dripping!" she told me. Apparently, she had not been able to make it stop.

I pointed out to her that the water was not on. Turning the faucet handle, I demonstrated the difference between on and off. I explained that the water left was simply that—water left as a lingering deposit from water that had been flowing through the hose at some earlier time. Of course, I thought confidently that I had taken care of the matter. However, she called my attention to the mouth of the hose again.

"But it's still dripping," she said.

SOURPUSS

Fri, 4 October 96

The mom seems to be in a rather dour mood tonight. I noticed this in her facial expression when I picked her up at daycare this evening. I asked what was wrong, and the owner of the facility said that one of the personnel had brought a large, very realistic-looking baby doll with her today. Apparently, my mom had insisted on holding the doll most of the day, but at one point she had told them that the baby was dead. Although they had told her over and over that it was a doll, she refused to buy it. I don't know why this has affected her as it has, but she has been really pigheaded tonight. A no-eat night and a general range of misunderstandings.

It's funny the way she can still come up with some of her ploys from her earlier, saner days. Although I'm sure it is entirely accidental, it seems a bit eerie at times. One of the annoying things she used to do in years gone by was that whenever we went on a trip, long or short, as we began to approach home on the return trip, she would begin to speculate about what had gone wrong at home in our absence. She would continue this on and on to such an extent that one would wish that one had not gone in the first place.

Back in 1983, when my parents had taken me with them to Galveston to see my daughter in an out-door drama, on the return trip my mom began when we were about two hours from home to do the agonizing-about-the-state-of-home thing. By the time we got there I was thoroughly fed-up to such an extent that even she realized that I was angry.

After I had gone to bed, she came in and sat on my bed and said that she didn't know what she had done to make me mad, but she hoped I'd forgive her. Now, that sounds good, but it wasn't really because she managed to say it in such a way as to lay the guilt and blame on me for having gotten annoyed. I realize now that she used the guilt-trip-application frequently.

Oddly enough, she suddenly pulled that out this evening after she had not eaten dinner, had mixed the potatoes and gravy with her hands, and had finally wondered plaintively if she might be permitted to go to the bathroom. She hoped that I wouldn't mind her going. Now, I had already taken her into the bathroom twice at what had seemed to be her request, with no result except for her becoming upset because I was trying to force her to do something she didn't want to do. All big-eyed, she said she hoped that I wouldn't have bad feelings about her for asking to be taken to the bathroom.

She takes Klonopin twice a day, but we have almost used all the current prescription. She will be seeing the doctor on Monday, but in the meantime, we're going to be doing a half tab a day. It looks to be a long weekend.

MY LITTLE RUNAWAY

Sat, 5 October 96

My son says that he can't tell that the Klonopin makes much difference. However, after today I can most definitely affirm that it makes a lot of difference. I've stayed with the mom on the weekends for the last month and a half, and having her take the med in the morning makes for a great difference in the day. I was wrong about having enough medication left to give a limited dosage all weekend long. There are two whole tabs left, and I figure that's one for Sunday evening and one for Monday morning.

It's important for her to have it before going to daycare. We don't want them to kick her out. It's not as if she were no trouble. Occasionally (Well, actually four times the daycare owner says.), they have missed the visible signs that she was thinking about defecating, and she got away before they saw her. Apparently, there is a closet she likes. A real mess resulting, I gather.

Normally, she naps a little from time to time, but today I think she stayed awake all day. For those who think that keeping her a little sedated is unkind—you should wonder whether it is beneficial to anyone to have a mindless automaton roaming around, purposeless, directionless, talking constantly, and moving everything she gets her hands on.

The high point of the morning came when I, having opened all the entrance doors to the house, thinking I had everything under control, became absorbed in drilling holes in order to install a hanging device in the kitchen. I suddenly realized that the mom was not on the back deck, and I discovered after looking all over the house and roaming the yard, front and back, yelling "Hortense!," that she was gone. So, it was get in the pickup and start looking.

She wasn't at my son's house, which is about two and a half blocks away, or in any of the immediate neighborhood. I finally found her in the park, picking up sticks and walking briskly eastward. The park is about six blocks away. I'm surprised she got there so fast.

I was not happy, and neither was she. So I double-locked all the doors for the rest of the day, but resented it, I'm afraid. A waste of good weather.

DRUG FREE MISERY

Sun, 6 October 96

What an incredibly horrible weekend! We are never, never, never (Keep repeating it!) going to run out of Klonopin on a weekend again. I can't even stand to think about it yet, much less write about it. Manana.

REMEMBERING

Tue, 8 October, 96

Perhaps it is because I have prided myself over the years for being patient and not exploding over things, that a tendency I am showing lately is very troubling to me. Actually, there is some humor in the situation if viewed from the proper perspective, which I don't seem to have at the moment. I don't think I am behaving too admirably at times like this past weekend.

Back when I was anticipating retiring and discussed it with people, I would mention my mother and say (Rather sanctimoniously, I guess.) that I had only one time to do this and wanted to do it right. That is hilarious! The way I have been behaving toward my mother is so far from even-tempered and patient that I should blush to remember my intentions. Right? Correctly or appropriately? I don't think so!

Maybe it's because I have a lot of stored up hostility that never was expressed. Dunno. I know that when I was growing up, I didn't particularly enjoy my mother's company. I can't remember wanting to spend time with her after my childhood and youth were past. In the grown-up years I have always dreaded having to go to visit.

However, in more recent years I managed to work my way around to feeling sympathetic for a lot of things that seemed to have happened to her over the years. We even bonded a little. On the other hand, since 1992 I have been taking yet another look at the past—trying to see how things really were and what happened—and have discovered that I probably didn't see things clearly at all when I was growing up. Therefore, I've moved away a bit from the more recent sympathetic stance.

A couple of anecdotes:

Back in the forties my father crushed a disk in his back and eventually had surgery for it, but in those days they handled it differently than they do now. It left him fused at that spot on the spinal column, unable to bend from the waist and suffering some pain over the years.

In the mid-sixties, he was the IRS officer in charge of Collections for north Mississippi and was riding in the car of one of his assistant workers who didn't have seat belts. A girl driving another car hit their car on the passenger side, injuring my father. He was taken to Memphis with a broken hip, broken ribs, punctured lungs, etc.

He eventually was sent back home to Water Valley, Mississippi to recuperate, using a wheelchair for his early convalescence. After a time he went back to work again on crutches and eventually discarded them, too. Unfortunately, his was one of those cases where the hip never healed. They put a pin in the hip, but that didn't work either. After a time, the pin broke, leaving gristle holding the joint together, or so I was told. Over time, one leg became shorter than the other, causing him to limp and generating some pain in his back and hip for the rest of his life.

On the brighter side, he was stationed in Jackson, Mississippi, and was able to complete study for and acquire his C.P.A. Also, because of the availability of night-time law classes there from the University of Mississippi, he was able to attend those and complete a law degree. He passed the bar exam, and in the early seventies, when he took his thirty years retirement, he was able to go back to Water Valley and practice law for about fifteen years.

Now, for a good part of this time, my mother had a remark she would make: "Well, you know, Dick is just a cripple."

I think my father had been very determined to marry her. He had regarded her as "his girl" since they were kids. I think he must have cared a good bit, if he were able to forgive her remark. So far as I know he never commented on it.

The second story:

Sometime back in the late forties, my father gave my mother a food mixer set for Christmas. They weren't as common in those days and so this was kind of special. It was a stationary mixer with bowls and attachments. This also was a time before it was universally recognized that appliances aren't appropriate personal gifts. I remember my mom opening the package and giving this plaintive little howl of disappointment. Something like" Oh, Noooooooooooo!" She has used that since then for numerous things.

The problem was, it seemed, that she had been eyeing a couple of women's suits at a clothing store in town. She was waiting to see them go on sale, hoping she could buy them. Now that I think back, I think she got them anyway. I'm pretty sure of that.

I have come to realize in these later years that the mom has had some unusual notions regarding money management. I wish I had paid more attention to what happened back then, but I was pretty much a "seen but not heard" kind of kid, which was not as unusual then as it is now. However, there wasn't really too much opportunity to be otherwise because the mom was an obsessive, continuous talker, and my paternal grandmother, with whom we lived, was no mean conversationalist either.

SELF-EVALUATION

Tue, 8 October 96

What I really hate is this propensity for violence I am beginning to see in myself. Over the weekend—on Sunday in particular—there were moments when I knew I could very easily, if I let myself go, completely waste the poor little woman. I have come to understand now why people abuse the elderly, and it is horrible that this is so. We're never going to be without the Klonopin again. I can deal with simple caretaking, but when the problem is complicated by the vestiges of her personality and compulsions, it is almost more than I can bear.

My son learned Sunday that a very good friend of his may have pancreatic cancer and may be dying. Sunday night, I couldn't help thinking about the irony and the waste in this situation, where this guy, who knows how to enjoy life and has a life, may be extinguished, while my mother and I, who serve no earthly purpose that I can see, go on and on and on.

Well, no one says that life is just.

GODIVA

Mon, 14 October 96

It's a strange thing (or maybe not) that often when one thinks that one has things in hand, it turns out that one is in error. It's been a good day, full of lawn mowing, window washing, etc. Progress! I had gotten stuff for dinner and had kind of a plan in mind. Well!

When I picked up the mom at daycare, the girl who brought her out told me that Mom had been a little more disoriented than usual today. She said that the mom had started taking off her clothes in front of the group. This is not a thing that bothers me much. Hey, I've bought her some new underwear, and she was wearing it!

We were a little late getting home because I stopped to buy some pansies and to get the mom some ice cream sandwiches, which I had forgotten to buy earlier. When we arrived at home she decided that she needed to go to the bathroom. Fine. Then she proceeded to entirely remove her red warm-up pants. I remonstrated, thinking that she would find it uncomfortable without them (She did.). In order to stop her from putting the pants in the trash, I took them to another room. When I returned she had removed her shoes and socks. Again I pointed out the unwisdom of this.

Eventually, we ended up in the kitchen, so that I could prepare something for us to eat. I finally fed her the meal spoonful by spoonful because she kept trying to put her food on her feet and ankles and calves. I'm afraid I didn't stay entirely calm. Of course, by that time she was complaining that she didn't have any clothes, and what should she do? She kept reaching for a bowl on the floor that I had used to feed one of the cats in the morning and had neglected to remove and clean. I think she was considering using it as a shoe. Who knows!

Moral: One should not get too chirky about how well one is dealing with things.

GOOD DRUGS

Wed, 15 October 96

Regarding Klonopin, the reason the mom has ended up taking it is because I was taking it for a while. For a few months, I was having great difficulties sleeping and needed something to enable me to sleep through the night, but I finally got past it. I don't think her present doctor (family practice) is particularly knowledgeable about treating psychological illness or about geriatric medicine. She's pleasant, attractive, and even-tempered—very much in control of her life. She also has more control than I have ever had or wanted to have, regarding food intake. She looked about five months pregnant when she was within a week or two of delivery, and then she managed to fit in the whole delivery thing and subsequent experience into one month, for which she had arranged a temporary doctor to sub. The well-ordered life. One wonders if it is always going to work that way. I would think not. Life tends to be untidy.

A related food store—the shorter of her two nurses told me that the doctor and her two nurses sometimes share a two-fer cookie pack from the vending machine. The taller nurse gets a whole cookie, but the doctor and the shorter nurse get a half cookie apiece. No danger of overdoing it!

One might wonder why the mom is not going to a geriatric specialist. Well, my son took her to a clinic in Birmingham—one that specializes in conditions like hers. Dementia, I suppose. They ran tests and intended to do one where they examined her hands to determine something or other, but it was not completed. As I understand it, what they planned to do was to use it to counsel me and my son so as to explain to us what we could expect in the future, and, perhaps, to help us work through our grief or something. Inasmuch as time was a limited commodity, and since we knew perfectly well what it was like to deal with her, we felt that it wouldn't be very useful.

With our current doctor, we tried a few drugs, one of which—Haldol—made her so antsy as to be unbearable. Tranquilizers were out because they would simply reduce her motor skills, although she would be just as impelled to move and get into things as usual. However, there would then be greater opportunity for injury.

Injury, naturally, is something to be avoided, since it seems that it never results in anything that would require hospitalization. This last sounds callous, but one finds that it is an attitude that one finally comes to. If she is hospitalized, then someone else is, momentarily, being paid to look after her. If not, one must do it oneself, and this is for a woman who usually has to be strapped in bed when she is in the hospital because she is determined to get up as soon as she wakes up. She can get very angry if she is not permitted to do so. Fortunately, she is not violent yet. However, I have seen enough hate in her eyes upon those few occasions when I lost my patience and picked her up bodily to put her in bed that I don't want to see her begin acting out those irritations.

ZOLOFT SPELLS HOPE?

Thu, 17 October 96

Well, the mom has been put on Zoloft for a three week trial period, 50 mg. a day, which, based on my own experience with Zoloft, seems like a low dose. I don't recall exactly, but it seems to me that I was taking 200 mg. a day at one time. Anyway—last night was very trying, but tonight, so far, is much better.

I think I have already written elsewhere on line about the time I fell into the channel behind the house and sent my mother to find and bring a ladder, but I don't think I've done anything definitive on the cat food. So!

In the spring of '93 when I brought my mother from Water Valley to Montevallo, she had on hand three cats and one dog, all quite elderly. The dog had a pronounced limp as a result of the mom hitting it with her car when she left home hurriedly back in the eighties. For the trip, I put the animals in three cat carriers and one big dog carrier, all of which I placed in the back of my pickup. The rest of the load consisted of coolers containing the contents of the refrigerators. With this cargo, we made the nearly-five hour drive across the better part of two states. What a great trip! I attempted to entertain the mom with tapes of things like "Joseph and the Amazing Technicolored Dreamcoat." She didn't seem to approve of that too much, but then, I guess she was even more anxious than I had realized. Certainly more than I had anticipated.

I suppose it was because she no longer had a family to look after and prepare for that she had come to attend her animals as if they were her family. Unable to distinguish clearly between cans of dog food and cat food (I really did try for a while to buy dog food, too.), she gave them all cat food. For a while she preferred chopping up wieners for them, but eventually she came down to providing them with a variety of cat food. It was her feeling, apparently, that they needed to be fed three times a day, and she liked to give them a variety at each meal—three or four cans each—which she usually stirred with her fingers, regardless of its state of freshness. One can go through a fair amount of cat food that way.

One of the cats was killed by roving dogs the first summer; another died of some kind of disease—possibly distemper—in the summer of '95. The other cat and the dog lasted until the winter of '95–'96. In the meantime, however, since my mom followed the animals around the yard, bringing the cans to the place where the animal was sitting or lying, there always seemed to be cans of semi-rotting cat food everywhere. A definite turn-off.

She also tried to give her own food—whatever was served her—to the animals. Most often she did. I have seen her serve them hamburger fragments, nuts, candies, pepper, shrubbery—a very strong-willed and independent woman in some respects.

It was because of the rapid turnover in cat food that I often would go to the local market and buy as many as 99 cans of cat food. I especially remember the time when I had bought only 60 or 70 cans and had left them in paper sacks in her kitchen while I went up the slope to my house to deposit my own groceries. I came back down to finish putting away her stuff and found that she was busily opening the poptops of the cat food cans. At that point she had already opened twenty-one cans.

I got a little distraught, I'm afraid. Twenty-one cans, which, if we put them in the refrigerator to preserve them, she would forget. There was a time when the refrigerator would have dozens of cans of cat food in it in varying stages of decay. This is not to mention the others she would stash around the house just to have on hand—especially in her bedroom.

I remember that back in Mississippi before she left, she would mix moist/dry cat food with the actual wet meat cat food, trying to tempt the palates of the pussies. I discovered when I was cleaning out the last of the stuff in the house in Mississippi that in her personal clothes closet she had stored about eight to ten containers of the mixture that she had put aside at some point. It was fairly desiccated by then, but still a little gamy.

At least now I feed the current cats. I guess that's progress of a sort.

AUTUMN IN THE AIR

Mon, 21 October 96

An autumn observation—I was sitting with my mother on the back deck Sunday morning, doing some mending while she snoozed and fretted (Every time she awoke.). Very peaceful—except for Mom's complaints—with cooler air, the sunshine, and the sounds and sights of the water over the old mill dam on the creek below.

There were a fair number of insects. I don't know what the actual name of the bug I have in mind is, but there is one that I think we used to call a "humble bee." That may not be accurate, or I may be misremembering. Anyway, it is striped, a little like a yellow jacket and a little like a bee, but it is harmless. It tends to land on one and walk around examining the territory and then fly away. Sometimes you have to encourage it to leave, but mostly I don't bother. They do no harm. They do have a tendency to walk around the edges or on the tops of the glasses of whatever beverage one may be drinking. This seems strange when the beverage in question is un-sugared. Maybe they just want liquid? I don't know.

Anyway, I was taking a sip from my glass of Diet Pepsi, when a small lump washed against my lips and then back inside the glass. I looked inside, and there, washed up near the rim, was what looked to be the corpse of one of the little insects. I was saddened and placed the little body in an old empty ashtray. Regretting its passing, I went on with my button sewing, but after a bit, I was surprised by what looked like a faint movement in the bug. Looking closer, I saw that it was true! It was still alive!

I moved it gingerly to a more open place, and it dragged itself into an upright position and eventually began working its wings. And it flew off! Amazing, I thought!

It seemed even more amazing when, after we had gone inside for lunch, I discovered the corpse of another bug down among the remains of the ice cubes in my glass, and it, too, proved to be alive. Apparently, insects are a lot more resilient than I ever thought. This particular kind, at least.

FURTHER EXPLORATION

Mon, 21 October 96

Well, I went to see my doctor today. My mother and I have both changed doctors, by the way. After we had engaged in some conversation she decided to let me try an anti-anxiety med called Buspar (Buspirone Hcl). Each tab contains 15 mg. and can be divided into as small an amount as a fifth, which is what I took at four P.M. today, and I must say that I have been much calmer. No rages, which is the way I like it. I hope it continues.

The shoe finally dropped this weekend while I lay down in the afternoon to rest a little and to ease some pain. My legs were aching—I suppose because of arthritis. Unfortunately, I briefly dozed off while I was waiting for my aspirin to take effect. Apparently, the mom awoke from her almost continual Saturday nap, took herself to the kitchen, and used the large wastebasket for a chamber pot.

Maybe it was the silence that roused me? Anyway, I suddenly came awake, listened for sounds and, becoming suspicious, went in search of the mom. Big mess in the middle of the floor. She was standing at the sink with the water running, wearing only her warm-up top, and was apparently attempting to clean up the mess with a sponge. She had closed the door into the room, which said something. Oddly enough she didn't get any excrement on her shirt, but she did get it everywhere else. We both were a little surly for a while. Probably, it was my fault to some extent for having given her some applesauce the night before. Live and learn.

It is kind of interesting that she has this ability to pick a time when I was out. She had been asleep when I lay down, and usually she nags at me whenever she is awake, but this time she made no sound and left me alone. It seems to me that there is something here of the puppy who, when annoyed with the owner, goes and makes a mess on the carpet.

Sunday morning was fairly quiet, though busy for me. When I finally took the mom out on the back deck where I sat and sewed some buttons back on a couple of her sweaters, she said that she wanted to go down the back steps and go back to Mississippi. After she had made a few attempts to go down the steps from the deck, I put the restraining jacket on her, which secured her to her chair, so then she napped, and I sewed.

In the afternoon we went out to the house I bought last October (1995), when I moved out of her house and let my son move in to take care of her. At the time, it looked as if he were going to be able to sell this house in which I now am living. However, that fell through, and so, in December, 1995, I moved back into this house.

Although I was able to rent out the house in Wilton, an immediately adjacent town, last December, and it has remained rented since then, unfortunately, my tenant moved out the 1st of this October, so we are scrambling trying to get it sold or rented.

Therefore, Sunday afternoon, I took my mother out there with me, so I could trim some of the grass the tenant had let grow up in the flower/shrubbery beds around the front of the house. Things went okay, it seemed, as Mom circled the house over and over, making remarks about things as she went. She disappeared from sight as she began another circuit of the house.

In the meantime, I decided I'd had enough, collected my tools and prepared to go home. I called the mom. No answer. I went around the house, and called again, this time switching to "Hortense." As a former speech teacher/amateur actress I can project very well. I'm sure everyone in the neighborhood heard me calling.

She wasn't answering, and I established that she was not in the barn nor in the house. Remembering how she had run off in the past, I got in the pickup, drove out to the highway and went down the road in both directions as far as she might be presumed to be capable of going. No luck.

So I went back to the house, mulling over possibilities and thinking to myself how fortunate it was that I had brought my usually useless cell-phone along. The house sits on four and a half acres of lightly timbered, heavily scrubby land—uneven terrain and footing. She had been having trouble seeing earlier in the day, and her footing has been unsteady for some time now. It was possible that she might have tumbled down one of the inclines and injured herself or hit her head on something.

So I started methodically from the lot in front of the barn again, yelling "Hortense" loudly at intervals. As I approached the downhill side of the barn, I saw her. She was in white warm-ups that day—quite visible, fortunately. Using a limb she had found as a walking stick, she was laboriously making her way up the slope. I yelled at her, but she didn't notice it at all. When we met, she remarked somewhat incoherently that she needed to pause because she was a little winded.

Small wonder! This is the woman who has been stumbling around the house for weeks, saying she couldn't see.

Of course it is inevitable that she is constantly having vision problems because of infections of her eyes and her eyelids. She rubs her eyes almost constantly, and this means that whatever she has touched with her hands, such as feces, leaves, or dirt, therefore gets rubbed on her eyes. It is a problem which has seemed impossible to control.

One bright spot—she didn't decide to wander in the other direction, which could have really produced problems. Well, I learned a valuable lesson. However cruel it might seem, unless I am going to be giving her all my attention when we are outside, I should always restrain her to a chair while we are outside. She can be gone in seconds, if she suddenly takes a notion to go, and there is no way of predicting it whatsoever.

Another bright spot: only about a week and a half remaining until she is back with my son for the weeknights for a month. I look forward to that. I had thought I'd be able to keep her all the time from now on. I was wrong.

TRIVIA

Wed, 23 October 96

The mom seems loathe to go to bed tonight. Not nearly as sleepy as usual, although she has received the same medications as usual tonight. This brings me to my first observation, which is that although the publications and literature on Alzheimer's lead one to expect a constant progression of deterioration, it isn't necessarily like that.

I remember that a couple of years ago, when the mom was not nearly as disoriented as she is now, she would suddenly pick up a ball point pen and try to eat with it. She also would choose paring knives for writing purposes. However, nowadays she frequently is still able to use a fork to eat with. She can distinguish the different foot shapes of shoes, oddly enough, and usually can pick the correct one for the foot she is intending to shoe. Not always, of course.

This time last year, one of the things that I found most wearing was the frenetic activity that my mom showed at the end of the day and toward bedtime, pacing from room to room, looking for God-knows-what and seemingly unable to settle down to go to bed. She was going to another daycare center then. The woman in charge told me it was typical of Alzheimer's victims and that it was called "Sundowning." I subsequently read about it in some of the literature. Getting her to bed used to drive me crazy. I remember, in particular, the Thanksgiving weekend in '95 that I spent with her. Much earlier I had picked rather bold patterned linens and a comforter for her bed—navy blue and white—thinking it might please her. I think the bold pattern was a mistake. She kept making and unmaking her bed. I would turn the bed down for her, and she would make it up again, and then I would turn it down again. I would suggest she go to bed. She would ask if there were a place where she could go. I would point out the bed and turn it down again. And so on.

I really lost it on the occasion of that Thanksgiving, I'm afraid, ending up bawling my head off. As usual, she just kind of looked at me, head cocked to the side a bit, a little like a watchful chicken. The Sundowning finally did get me down to such an extent that I couldn't stand it any more.

In some respects she is much easier to deal with now. She is still not entirely accustomed to my house, so she has a tendency to follow me around a lot, especially after a daycare day.

One of the reasons it was difficult in earlier years to be sure just what was wrong with her was her ability to "confabulate." For a long time, this helped her to avoid exposing her inability to answer some questions. When pinned down, of course, it became clear that she didn't know obvious things, such as her birthday or the current day. I suppose this was because she always was such a vocal person and had a decent vocabulary. She still has the ability to sometimes come up with phrases that can sound momentarily as if she knows what she is talking about.

I think she has fooled her younger brother to some extent. He is in his seventies and sits her occasionally on Saturdays. I suppose it is rather difficult for him, recognizing that he is the last of the family, or, rather, that he is going to be the last. I think, however, he may be finally seeing how things are. Still, I'm sure it's hard. He thinks he has fond memories, or, at least, he thinks fondly of them. I, on the other hand, do not remember life with my mother fondly.

She was always, I now realize, a very self-absorbed woman and thought of me as an extension of her life. I remember when I was 18, home from college for the summer, and I had started smoking in January. There was a part of a pack of Kools in my purse that I had not concealed further because it did not occur to me that I need worry about having my possessions searched. She did, however, and asked me what the cigarettes were doing in my purse.

At the time my father had been smoking since his college days. Finally, he sat down with me and said that he was sorry, but it just wasn't acceptable for girls to smoke. It was upsetting my mother, and he didn't want to see her upset. He said that he would stop smoking in order to encourage me to stop. And he did, so far as I know! I, on the other hand, only stopped briefly, and I continued to smoke for nearly 26 years.

It was my feeling that they didn't want me to stop because they were worried or concerned about me, but, rather, because my mother felt it reflected poorly on her.

Well, that was long ago. It would seem, however, if I can still bring it up that I may, even yet, resent it a bit. About time I got over it, what?

TRIVIA, TOO

Tue, 29 October 96

This evening, after dinner, as I was administering nighttime medications, I noticed that my mother's whitish gray warm-up pants were yellowed in streaks down the insides, leading me to the conclusion that she must have simply let go at some point during the day. Awfully yellow though. I had noticed the other day that her urine was rather dark. I suppose this must be because she cannot remember to drink adequate amounts of water.

Well, I have to take her to see the doctor on Friday morning to discuss her Zoloft, the samples of which will be finished next week. I can't see that it is making a big difference. She certainly was sufficiently argumentative and unpleasant this past weekend. However, it's mostly in the afternoon, so it may be a cyclic thing. Maybe an increase in dosage might help.

We stopped her anti-agitation medication after the last visit because the doctor pointed out that it was in the same family as Haldol, and, God knows, Haldol turned her into a real squirrel when she took that. That might explain some of her behavior the first weekend, when she was out of Klonopin, and I was giving her the other medication, thinking it might reduce her frenetic activity.

Anyway, there's a good bit of laundry to do these days. One of the things that Mom seems to have forgotten how to do, or to give any thought to doing in the first place, is to wipe herself after urinating or defecating. Makes for messy underwear at the best of times. I think I'm going to have to buy a couple of cheap packs of briefs tomorrow at the dollar store because it has been more practical lately to simply throw away her soiled underclothes. Unfortunately, it's not as easy to remove the dried excrement from her bottom that has accrued by the end of the day. It's also painful to her.

Same old same old. However, come Sunday night, I'll have the house to myself for a few days.

SMALL REVELATION

Wed, 30 October 96

As I was driving back from delivering the mom to daycare just now, I suddenly realized that I had something to be grateful for regarding my mother. This came as I looked across the median at all the bumper to bumper traffic going in to Birmingham and then at all the traffic around me heading into Shelby County. At least I have retired from my job. I imagine that if I had to get up, feed, wash up the mom (Apparently another bowels/clothing accident last night, and some really messy legs to be washed this morning.), get her dressed, and then, with the stench of fecal matter in my nostrils, get myself dressed for a day of work and drive in to Sunshine Manor, it would seem a great deal less cheery to me.

There are lots of people who have relatives in the Manor who seem to be employed. I think that would be more strain than I could easily deal with at the moment. I am grateful, indeed. Now, if I can just manage to remember that.

INJURY

I omitted mention in my original posts of what happened on November 1 to incapacitate me for the whole of that month and on through December. On Friday, November 1, after having gone to see my doctor, I returned to Montevallo, and since my regular service station was closed because of the death of the owner's brother—the funeral was that day—I went out to the BP station just south of town. I pumped my own gas, blithely headed in to pay my bill, and tripped on the curb just before getting to the door.

The woman ahead of me was holding the door open, fortunately. Otherwise, I probably would have hit my head on the door, whereas I only bounced my forehead on the doorsill as I sprawled full-length. I seemed to have taken most of the fall on my right arm and shoulder. Very painful. This was an event that colored the whole next month and lingered on for many months to come in small ways. I could hardly sleep at night at first and tending my mom that weekend—dressing, feeding, and bathing her—was painful, indeed.

DOWN-TIME

Mon, 11 November 96

I had last week off, but I spent this past weekend with the mom at my son's house. In all honesty, I think she is a little easier to manage at my son's house, but, then, she has lived there—except for the last month—since April, '93, so it should seem more familiar to her. Also he has a large screen TV and full cable service (except for movie channels), whereas I became livid with Marcus Cable and canceled my service, leaving me with three VHF channels I pick up with rabbit ears. Actually, the reception is better now than what I was getting via cable. Anyway, the point is that there are more means of engaging her attention to some extent at my son's house.

I picked her up at daycare Friday evening, and we went directly to my son's house. She slept a good bit during the weekend. At one point on Sunday, while I was doing some housework, she started moving objects around. At the time, I was attempting to change the linens on the bed I was using during the visit, and her activity was interfering some, so I asked her to desist. I'm afraid I hurt her feelings. She then went into her bedroom and started moving her blankets. I figured she was going to take them off and fold them. Folding and stacking are seemingly constant involuntary activities with her. However, after a period of quiet, when I looked in to check on her, I discovered that she had crawled under the covers and was asleep. I imagine that in the midst of rearranging the bed-clothes, she lost track and thought she was going to bed. Anyway, after a lengthy earlier morning nap, she then slept for a couple of hours, right through lunch time.

One of the things I had dreaded in anticipation of the weekend was the aspect of potty-training. She had been moved from the largest bedroom in the house, with adjoining bathroom (again the largest) to a smaller room and a potty-chair. Unfortunately, she hasn't seemed to adjust to the chair yet. My son had told me that when he went in to get her Friday morning, he discovered her wearing only her shirt, with urine and feces all over the floor and fecal matter smeared on the walls. He asked me to encourage her to use the potty chair over the weekend. I could see his point.

Shortly after I got her home Friday night, she complained of stomach pain. It's very difficult to determine what causes her physical distress or where the cause is. Frequently, when I take her to the bathroom, it turns out that it wasn't really what she wanted, and we both get annoyed. If I make her sit down on the toilet—and she always wants to turn up both lids—she says I'm killing her. Of course, she also says this about baths. Apparently, this is typical of Alzheimer's victims. This time, however, it turned out she had diarrhea. No Immodium or other similar product in the house that I could find, so we went uptown (up the hill, actually) and bought some. No problems thereafter.

I don't know. It seems to me we may be in a new stage, but I could be wrong. Much more fuzziness, although she still has the impulse to get moving every time she wakes up and to begin talking. I guess lifelong compulsive talkiness doesn't die easily. She has confabulated for so long. She still does, uttering sentences with great conviction, but very often the words of emphasis will be nonsense words. However, since she doesn't understand the sense of one's response, I don't suppose it matters.

TERMS OF ENDEARMENT I

Tue, 19 November 96

Ever since the movie *Terms of Endearment* came out, and I read somewhere what the title referred to, the concept has stayed in my brain's current-stuff file to be pulled out and pondered a little from time to time. If there are those who are unaware, as I was, of what's being referred to, it is not words of endearment, but, rather, periods or phases. My son was mentioning when he returned from their lake house Sunday afternoon, as he was using the Sunday paper's sports sections to work up the results of his group's "You Pick 'Em" pool, that he was getting a little tired of doing it. He thought he was going to stop after this season. This brought to my mind the terms concept. Another enthusiasm had passed its peak.

TERMS OF ENDEARMENT II

Tue, 19 November 96

I hit the post button unintentionally, so that the last message was posted before I had finished. Then, after I started another message and had nearly completed it, Alabama Power had another of its little outages and—zap! Message gone! So time has elapsed since I wrote the last one. My usage of the terms of endearment reference was really intended to be applied more to family relationships than to a football pool. I think we all probably experience these phases in our lives.

This morning I would have written that I thought my mother was entering another stage and that she might soon be very nearly bedridden. Ha! I guess it was the cold she had this past weekend that rendered her so weak and unsteady yesterday, but she was definitely stronger tonight, with evidences of the old assertiveness. Still, she is getting thinner. She doesn't eat enough. The body obviously is burning muscle tissue, although she doesn't get around nearly as much, so that physical activity is not as big a factor as in the past.

All the literature I have read about Alzheimer's states that a point comes when they begin to lose their motor skills. I think we may be approaching it. One thing is for sure—she seems to have lost conscious knowledge of and control of the urination process, which will have to be dealt with. We are going to try those pads for incontinence.

TURN-OVER

Wed, 27 November 96

The first of December is rapidly approaching, and the time for moving the mom back to my house. Tomorrow is Thanksgiving, and I'm going to stay with her for it at my son's house. He has been working on a heating/cooling unit installation and has run into a snag, so he'll be working in the morning and then going with his girlfriend out to his dad's and stepmother's house on Lay Lake for Thanksgiving dinner. I think my daughter is going too, but the older son from Georgia and his family aren't going to be showing up this time.

Well, I'm a vegetarian, so the traditional Thanksgiving fare is out, but the mom still has to be fed, although she seems to be very limited in her tastes these days. Probably, I'll open a can of ravioli for her and maybe cook myself some black-eyed peas or butterbeans. Or I can heat an artificial soybean chicken pattie and make a sandwich. It doesn't really matter too much.

I bought a box of adult diaper pants today that I thought I would try out on the mom this weekend. I'm going to stay at my son's house with her, at least through Sunday afternoon, at which point, I'll move her to my place. She's been falling down a lot lately. I had begun to think that she might be bed-ridden by the time she got up here, but I observed when bringing her home tonight, that while unsteady, she was more herself. More assertive, more quarrelsome, more explorative.

Back around Monday, she fell on her face again. I know my son is scared to death that someone's going to think that he's abusing her. The truth is that he is much more patient and long-suffering than I. Of course, she's not his mother, either, which makes a difference. The trouble is, as long as she is insistent on moving when and where she wants to and as long as she becomes weaker and less sure of her balance, the more likely it is that she will take spills. On the other hand, as she becomes less assertive and more needing of personal care, the easier it is to take care of her.

I put some shelving across the lower part of the window in the room where she's going to be staying. I think this room will be easier to move in than the one where she stayed last time, and access to the bathroom is easier—no dog-leg in this one. The reason for the shelving was because when I looked at the lower half of the window (which is one of those tall old-fashioned ones) with the venetian blind removed, I realized that the single pane of glass might prove vulnerable. Probably not, but there could be a fall of over ten feet down onto the air conditioning units below. Better safe than sorry, so I nailed two sections of that white enameled metal shelving flat against the window. It doesn't have to be terribly strong. Just strong enough to deflect her, if she goes stumbling in that direction. I still need to attach the hinges of a door in one doorway and put up three sets of hooks and eyes on doors. It's amazing. In addition to the closet door, there are 4 doorway entries into the room. I'm blocking up two of them, leaving access through the bathroom door and the door into the kitchen.

Well, enough of writing about all that!

PREP TIME

Fri, 29 November 96

I'm taking a break just now. The door is hung now, but since it wasn't there when I repainted the room last winter, it is still the color that my friend/tenant painted it back in '89—flat black—which, in a light-almond colored room, will very likely get the mom's attention. People at daycare tell me that often Alzheimer's patients lack depth perception, so that placing a dark colored mat at exits tends to keep them inside. It looks bottomless to them. So I wonder if the door is going to be horrifying to her?

My alcoholic, schizophrenic, gay friend who occupied this side of the house for a couple of years was about twenty-three when he moved in—still full of youthful exuberance—and he immediately painted all the woodwork in the front two rooms black. This door is the only thing left that color. I must admit that when I was painting and realized that he had also painted the framework holding up the suspended ceiling tiles black as well, I cursed a little. A lot actually. I guess I'll have to do something about the remaining door.

The mom was having some trouble walking yesterday, favoring her right leg. My son said that the day care folks were suggesting that she might have broken her hip. It seems unlikely to me, but I've been standing ready today to throw the wheel chair in the truck, in case they called and suggested that she be taken to X-ray.

Anyway, I think I'm going to stay at my son's with her this weekend. For one thing, it's on flat land, instead of on a hill. If we're doing the wheelchair bit, it will be much easier—less physically taxing for me. Also I haven't quite tended to everything in preparation yet. If my uncle sits with her tomorrow morning and early afternoon, I'll be able to come back here and clear the old driveway route so as to be able to drive my truck up next to the north side of the house.

Well. There are also some hooks and eyes that still need installing.

PONDERING

Sat, 30 November 96

Saturday—all day—and at the moment approaching noon here in the central time zone. I'm taking a rest from clearing old gardening trash off the old driveway, and I seem to have picked up a few fire ants in the process of clearing. I wonder why it is they can't just jump off or crawl off the body instead of creeping under the clothing and taking a bite. I may be taking a shower sooner than I intended.

It's raining lightly today, so I'm not sure I'm going to complete the task. High wet grass. Another thing—some of the protected spots are now bare ground, which, with rain, spells mud. Not a pretty prospect. I really should put some gravel on it, which, fortunately, I have on hand—a nice pile of pea gravel. However, those of you who have spread gravel by hand occasionally will know why I'm dogging this. Gravel is heavy anyway and spreading wet gravel in the rain is not a thing one seeks out for fun. Well, at least some of us don't.

I took the mom by the emergency room of the county hospital last night after picking her up at daycare. They X-rayed and found nothing wrong. This says a lot for the good old-fashioned diet and upbringing. Your average eighty-three year old woman could not fall as often as this woman does and not sustain bone injury. I've been using the wheel chair yesterday and today to transport her any distance of more than a few steps. With my current shoulder problem, I am just not capable of supporting her full body weight for more than a very short distance. A great deal of the problem arises from her tendency to want to move. Often. Because she cannot remember causes and consequences, whether she is well or unwell, she craves perpetual motion. When she has mended from a fall and can kind of walk again, she will once again embark on a walk and will eventually lose her balance and fall down a few times.

This morning I brought her in the wheelchair into the kitchen to eat. Having accomplished that, I told her to stay exactly where she was while I got her clothes, which are kept in the guest bedroom. Therefore, I was just across the room from her when she decided to get up. I told her to sit down. She took a step or two and sprawled. I guess I should have put the confining jacket on her. Not thinking ahead, I guess. I told her to stay there until I got to her. Did she? No! She started crawling across the floor in the direction of the kitchen, moaning as she went.

Sometimes, however, she does pay attention to what you tell her to do. At others, it means nothing at all. Her only world seems to be inside her head and is concerned with what she thinks she is going to try to do. Or, maybe, it's a matter of a pattern of random impulses that move her accordingly.

I did, at least, move nearly all her clothes up here, so the move tomorrow should be fairly simple except for the problem of transport into the house.

DEPRESSION

Sat 30 November 96

Possibly, just how depressed an individual gets when tending an Alzheimer's victim may depend on how prone they were to depression earlier in their lives. Unfortunately, I have been depressed sometimes earlier in my life, turning my feelings inward upon myself. There were a couple of occasions after my divorce in 1978, when a low dose of anti-depressant was prescribed for me for brief periods. However, I didn't get into longish-term medication until the spring of '93 when I moved the mom from northwest Mississippi to Montevallo. Shortly thereafter, at the same time I began treatment for carpal tunnel syndrome, I started on Prozac, went to Zoloft, and finally settled on Paxil, with non-medicated periods at intervals.

When I read the drug records of the people who used to post in the mental health folders online and saw the combinations of drugs they took, I realized how fortunate I have been in that respect. My life has not been perfect, any more than most people's have. Something seems to have happened in my early years, around four to six that has affected me profoundly, so as to cause me to disbelieve and distrust professions of other people's affection for me and to avoid physicality like the plague. However, I know of so many people who have absolutely wretched lives that I realize I'm fortunate by comparison! I have survived life, although the periods with my mother over the years have always been down-times for some reason.

I am not on medication for depression at the moment. I'm not deeply clinically depressed right now, although I am taking Vasotec for hypertension, Glucophage and Glucotrol for diabetes, and an over-the-counter painkiller for my shoulder and arm. However, it is very easy to lose sight of any kind of positive outlook when you are dealing with a not-very-well-liked Alzheimer's patient.

Unless one has planned financially, it can seem as if all the family resources are being expended to extend the vital signs for a walking, stumbling, madwoman. If a family has any money—if the patient has a good bit of money—it can be very expensive providing care. Lacking enough money, but with too much to easily qualify for federal aid, then the family will have to expend its own time and energies on caregiving. This may require constant supervision, so that the patient doesn't wander off into traffic, into a stranger's house, or to the other side of town. These things happen to the patients and their caregivers all the time. All the time.

Caregivers are human. I think that even the best of us—which I am not by any means—have times when we wonder if we are going to have any life left when it is all over. I used to wonder if I would ever get over agonizing about the imperfections of the way I have handled this. I know now that I will be able to go on, but the problem right now is that one can't really believe that the ordeal will ever be over. One's own life comes to seem absolutely pointless because it is being expended in a seemingly pointless enterprise.

Occasionally, I think that I wish that I could die, but I couldn't kill myself because I can't leave this problem of my mother to fall entirely on my younger son. That would be unfair. Besides, my business affairs are in such a mess that I can't just leave them that way. So through sheer laziness, or maybe because I don't really want to give up whatever possibilities life may yet hold, I hang on. I know there are many, many people out there very much like me, who must wonder daily what they have done in their lives that was so bad, that they must pay for it in this coin. Irrational, of course, but it's hard to remember that it is irrational. I have had a month of relative freedom, but throughout the time, there was the knowledge in the back of my mind that the time was limited and that my world was once again going to shrink to a cave where the primo activities were spoon-feeding the mom so that she could maintain strength to go on living and falling down, and cleaning her ass on a daily basis after her fecal accidents.

I didn't really dislike my mother when this began. It has taken several years to bring me here.

ON THE ROAD AGAIN

Sun, 1 December 96

Move completed! As I expected, when I attempted to drive the pickup around the old driveway, once it hit the muddy parts, it bogged down. Fortunately, I was able to back up. Therefore, I had to wrestle the wheelchair around from one side of the house to the other.

Not a good night. Mom woke me about 2 A.M., apparently having decided to take off her pajama bottoms and diaper. It may be that she wanted to use the bathroom. Impossible to tell. Anyway, she went back to bed and, apparently, to sleep. I, on the other hand, didn't sleep for a great while. I thought about a lot of things.

I have decided to sell off everything except the bare essentials—or even give the stuff away if necessary. Why have two TVs if you only watch two or three shows a week? Simplification!

Mom woke me about 6 A.M., and this time she was taking off her clothes in earnest. Apparently, it really was for urination this time. I assisted her in stripping down, and then she went back to bed. A strange day. I'm very tired and sleepy.

I figured out I couldn't kill me or my mother because both of our pensions are needed to keep family finances afloat at the moment—that is, the financial situation that has been brought into being through bringing Mom over here.

WHEELCHAIRS

Thu, 5 December 96

When my father broke his hip back in the mid-sixties, he bought a wheelchair that he used for a while during his recuperation. Toward the end of his life, in the mid-eighties, he used it again. After his death the chair was stored, and we brought it over to Alabama in 1993 with all the other household goods. Thank goodness we did! However, I must say it seems to be a fairly heavy model, and I say this as a person who lifts things pretty well.

This is another little world we are exploring and learning about. One of the things that drives me absolutely crazy about wheelchair transport is the mom's tendency to drag her feet or brace them against the upcoming pavement or ground. One asks what is the matter—sometimes irately, depending on the time of the day and what's been happening—and discovers she has her feet braced against the hillside. Thus, the pusher of the wheelchair and she are laboring against one another.

I noticed the manager at the daycare center avoids that by raking the chair upward. I, however, at the end of the day, am pushing her uphill halfway around the house through grassy, stubbly turf. By the time we have made it even to the front of the house—which has two flights of steps down to the street, not to mention a set of steps leading up to the porch—I am getting bushed. I begin to appreciate the concept of ramps.

Oh, well. I daresay I will learn something from the experience. (Actually, I did, and by the time she was back down at my son's house, I had become fairly adept at pulling the chair backward up steps.) I don't know whether she's going to walk again or not. Sometimes it's hard, just getting her to stand up. I think I've got to be more careful of my back when trying to move her. Otherwise, I could end up with severe injury.

NEW STAGE

Sun, 8 December 96

I'm not sure just where we are. When I arrived at daycare on Friday evening they said that the mom had been groggy all day and that she'd had an accident. Inasmuch as I'd put her in diapers that morning, and they had replaced both her socks and pants, I suspected she might have had diarrhea. I think I was in error about that, however. They asked if I had given her anything extra that morning so as to cause increased drowsiness, but I had not. Still, I noticed that she drooped over in the car seat, nearly doubled over, even with the seat belt and harness fastened. This worried me a bit, and since she had been so hard to get on her feet when putting her in the car and because I thought she might have a bug or have had a little stroke, I decided to stop at the county hospital emergency room on our way home. After all, it wasn't as if anyone was waiting for us to get home, so it didn't really matter where we spent the evening.

It turned out to be nothing in particular. They contacted her/my doctor, who suspected she was over-medicated. At the time I was a bit offended by this, but now that we have almost completed the weekend, I think that may have been true to some extent. That is true in terms of what seems to be her current state. I remember well how in August of 1995, I came down to cook her breakfast and discovered that she couldn't keep her face out of her food. This has happened a time or two since then, and I guess this latest was simply another instance.

I didn't bring her to my home Friday night because I didn't think I could keep her in the wheelchair all the way around the house or, for that matter, even lift her into the wheelchair in her current state. Anyway, we went to my son's house—he'd gone to the lake—to spend the night It's on flat ground, and there are only a couple of flat stones leading up to the back porch. Mom was a little more aware by then, so we made it inside fairly well. I did give her half a Klonopin and her Zoloft that night, but I have given her no more Klonopin since then.

I don't think she was awake more than 2 or 3 hours at the very most on Saturday. Part of this was spent sitting up in a chair; the rest, in bed. When she attempted to stand, she couldn't do it without help, and it required a lot of bracing on my part. She was awake in bed for a while this afternoon, so she will probably sleep tonight. Anyway, I'm now sleeping in a single bed in her bedroom, so I awake whenever there is any noise.

I think this is a new stage. It seems as if her body has forgotten how to maintain the upright stance. While I was sitting in the room at emergency looking at her on the bed, I suddenly became aware of how much she has deteriorated since September. Only two months ago, she ran away to the park. Somehow, I don't think she could do that now, even if I never gave her any Klonopin again. One of the doctors on duty remarked that she was in the late stages of Alzheimer's and that she needed to be in a nursing home. I explained about the money situation, and that was that.

I think this is one of those periods of sudden deterioration. One feels a bit strange about this. I wish I had been pleasanter, but I don't think I could have managed it. Guess I'll have to try harder now.

FLASH

I was driving downtown on some errands a while ago, feeling kind of down and weepy, when it suddenly hit me what part of my problem is, and, probably, from whence some of my rage derives. I am neither a registered nor practical nurse. I have received no training in such a field. In addition, I have no experience nor training for dealing with people with senile dementia of whatever origin or with the insane. I think what I was feeling last night, as I peered into the semi-darkness and saw the surreal spectacle of my mother swinging around—careening around—the bed posts, was a feeling of utter helplessness and hopelessness, in addition to the experience of disorientation. When I had gotten her back to bed, with no real hope of her remaining there, wondering if I was going to sleep again before dawn—what I was feeling was despair and desperation because I am not really competent to deal with that which must be dealt with.

There have been so many things in my professional life that I was expected to lie about and pretend to be—to be a trained costumier and costume designer, for example, which I was not and had no real desire to be. In those days I was such a great fool that I didn't have the sense to call a halt and declare that I was not the role I was trying to play. I think this is more of the same and that what is happening here is kind of a "last straw" effect, in terms of pretending to be competent at what I'm not. I think part of the rage stems from that. Role-playing stretched to the limit

My God, I hope she is manageable tonight, or that I reach a stage of peace or numbness before then! What does one do with an active madwoman in one's own home? Besides feed her and keep her clean? I haven't a clue!

TODAY

Tue, 10 December 96

At one o'clock this morning, I woke and saw that Mom was out of bed standing at the doorway to the bathroom. As I watched she lost her balance and fell. At the emergency room they discovered that she had, indeed, broken her hip this time. It's a clean break, however, where the leg bone joined the hip bone socket. They did surgery late this afternoon and put in a pin. They're expecting to start rehab tomorrow. She'll probably be in the hospital a while for this.

I have mixed feelings. I had bought a lot of rope yesterday for the purpose of tying her in the wheelchair and into the bed if needed. If I had used the rope to make bed restraints for her, would she have fallen? I'll never know.

I feel very bad for my uncle, her younger brother, who is in his mid-seventies. He joined the air force during World War II and was shot down over the African desert. He spent the rest of the war in prison camp in Germany. He can verify all the tales from *Hogan's Heroes* and *Stalag 13*, except that they weren't comedies, but deadly serious. One doesn't think of him as being particularly old. Obviously, he's a good bit younger than my mother—the youngest member of the family.

Anyway, his wife was telling me at the hospital that he sometimes sits at home and says—referring to his says—"She's all I've got left."

POST-OP

Wed, 11 December 96

The mom had a good night, they say, so I imagine they had her sedated. I was told that they had her sitting up for two hours this morning. When I got to the hospital this afternoon, my aunt and uncle were there with her. She doesn't have a private room, so I can't help feeling a little sorry for patients who have to share the room with her.

The nurses had given her a suppository, and she was strenuously and vocally, though incoherently, resisting the effect of the suppository. This offered an opportunity to observe just how agitated she can become, how strong she can be, and just how much she needs constant supervision if left unmedicated. I stayed to feed her the evening meal. By that time they had given her some anti-agitation medication, although they are still in the process of finding a medication that is truly effective.

In my opinion, the restraints they have on her wrists are far too long. She had already pulled something loose on one wrist shortly after I got there. I intend to return for the lunchtime meal tomorrow. It looks as if she's going to be in for a while for hospitalization and for rehab. There is something a little bizarre about expending so much energy and money on rehabilitating a woman who lacks understanding of where one might go or what might be done when one has arrived there. Ironic.

CHRISTMAS DAY

Wed, 25 December 96

My mother is being released tomorrow. Frankly, I think there must be a mix-up on this, but since my/her doctor is on vacation, there is not much to be done about it. I think that maybe my doctor suggested after-Christmas as a release time, and that the case worker seized on the day after Christmas, but I won't know for a while whether my guess is correct.

The case worker has given me some trouble, in my opinion, although I imagine she thought of it as merely going about her duty. She kept badgering me about selecting a nursing home. In response, I suggested that we might not be able to put Mom in a home, asking what would happen then. She stated that there were home health care options that might kick in then.

Finally, after a nursing home in a community up above Bessemer called, I made an appointment to go see the facility. It seemed nice, but after Mom's Medicare was exhausted, the facility would charge $97 a day, exclusive of meds and additional stuff. $97 X 30 = $2910, which is more than the total of the mom's monthly pensions and her annuity. We are already pretty strapped, as it is. I imagine that the cost of this one was about as low as one could expect. When I consider what it's like to tend patients like my mother, I consider $97 a day fairly cheap.

As it turned out, the trip was in vain because their one available space had already been taken. In addition, it had snowed the day before, and there was a fair amount left on the roads to the north. Ever since my accident back in 1968 I haven't driven on snowy roads with any degree of pleasure. I wasn't a happy camper.

I have dropped by the hospital nearly every day, and nearly every time she was sitting up. She no longer blinks all the time or rubs her eyes. Instead, she stares, owl-like. They seem to have finally gotten her agitation under control, and let me tell you, she had SOME agitation at times. At various times she has pulled out her catheter, the IV feed, and the telephone, and has also pulled off her night gown and her hand restraints. Some of these she has thrown at the nurses.

I remember being there one day when she was sitting in the chair alongside the bed, a sheet tying her to the chair, with her eyes closed, busily working at untying her hand restraints. They hadn't found an effective anti-agitation drug at that time. The nurse in the room looked at her, kind of sighed as she watched her undo one of the restraints with her eyes closed, and said in a strangled tone of voice: "She's good!"

It is understandable that they will be happy to see her go. One nurse told me brightly that her bed sore was much better and almost gone. Of course, I didn't know she had a bed sore.

As I understand it, the E.C.U. will not keep the mom for the additional time we had expected because of the psychiatric elements—she requires additional care—and the psychiatric unit wouldn't take her because of the broken hip—again, additional care. She mostly seems to be sitting up, so we are planning on sending her back to daycare next Monday, unless the next few days show that it can't be done. I must admit I am not looking forward to these next few days. I seem to have a mild bug of some sort—low grade temp, nausea, dizziness, occasional diarrhea—which will not help things.

I remember a time in the late eighties when my departmental chairman (my ex-husband) had suggested that I begin costuming one show per semester—returning to costuming again. At that time I went out to walk/run in the early morning. As I went, I would try to figure out how I was going to get through it all that day. Needing to choose a path to follow for the work that day, knowing I could not finish, but wanting to pick a way that would bring me closer. Lots of despairing mornings. Often I would think thoughts like: please, may I not let this cup pass from me? Do I absolutely have to do this?

I find myself thinking that kind of thing a lot lately. It may be just because I'm under the weather, but one does wonder what will be enough. When will one have sacrificed or suffered enough? Not just me. My son and his girl friend, also. And her, too. Definitely her, too. In her right mind, she would not choose this, even if it does make her the center of attention, which she has always loved.

Well, nothing to be done, but to do it, so tomorrow afternoon I will bring her home again, and we'll try to make it work until she can get up and fall and injure herself again. I understand that happens a lot with people like her.

NEW YEAR'S DAY

Wed, 1 January 97

One week later. Tomorrow, when I pick up the mom at daycare, I'll be taking her to my son's house. Things haven't been so bad, although I've continued to run a low grade fever and have felt kind of lousy a lot of the time, which has made picking her up and dressing her very exhausting. I usually have to take a break during the process.

She now has two medicines that she has to take daily: 1) Digoxin C-5 mg—for her heart, and 2) Loxapine Hydrochloride—5 ml four times a day for agitation.

Her incision was nicely healed when she came home, and they have had her walking a bit at daycare. In fact, yesterday evening, when I got her home, she wanted to go on walking—staggering around. Now I daresay there are those who would say: let her go! There certainly are advantages to having her able to stand up. It makes dressing her much, much easier. However, the more she roams, the more room there is for accident. Anyway, by the time I had wrestled the wheelchair around the house in the dark to the sidedoor, feeling unwell, I wasn't much in the mood for an exercise session. Anyway her diaper and the seat of her sweats were pretty wet, so she needing changing.

What a strange life this seems to be! Maybe I'll think differently about it when I'm feeling better again? However, it may be a good thing I'm scheduled to see my therapist tomorrow.

THE BEAT GOES ON ...

Sat, 4 January 97

I think going to talk to the therapist was a good thing, although I hated to spend the money. I hadn't been to see her since September. At that point I was only anticipating beginning the alternation of months of keeping the mom. I was only getting ready then to move her in for October, so I had lots and lots to discuss. It was kind of nice to have someone tell me that I had done okay. I suppose one should know this for oneself, but this isn't a strength of mine. Too much dependence on outside sources for verification of my having succeeded, regarding some things.

Well, I think every inch of my house and yard needs attention of some sort, and I am still running a low grade fever and suffering some kind of intestinal thing for part of each day. It slows one down and saps the will. I guess I need to see my doctor next week, although I can't imagine what could be done to help much. I never seem to get sick enough from transient things to have stuff prescribed. Well, that's not quite true. When I stepped on the roofing nail in 1994, I got to take quite a lot of good stuff before we finally tamed the infection.

I stopped by my son's house to leave a magazine early this afternoon. The mom was sitting in the wheelchair in the living room in front of the TV. She looked mildly hostile, but, apparently, she isn't giving too much trouble. He is discovering that it is necessary to confine her some at night in order to keep her in bed and avoid reinjury. I was afraid that this was going to be the case when she recovered a bit more. I had tied her in the last two nights she was here.

STATUS

Wed, 15 January 97

Well, the mom seemed to suffer a little spell a few days ago and has spent much of her time since then leaning out of the wheelchair to her right, with her eyes closed, seemingly barely conscious of being alive. My son said he was having trouble getting her to eat and that she was assuming a kind of fetal position in bed at night.

However, she seems to be recovering a little again, sitting up straight, keeping her eyes open most of the time and able to hold a glass at times. This doesn't mean that she's making a recovery, of course. She's still in the wheelchair and has to be nearly lifted from it into and out of the truck.

I'm to see my doctor tomorrow. I've been running a low grade fever since before Christmas, and I have no desire at all to get up in the morning or to stay up, once I'm up. It's pretty certain I'm depressed. Lordie! I would love to wake up with enthusiasm for the day again someday. It's been a long time since that happened, but at least my attitude was a little better back in November and early December.

PUREE

Wed, 22 January 97

I just returned from bringing the mom back home from the day care facility, and I can't help thinking she has lost more ground in some ways. Hard to pinpoint, but still there is that sense.

Last weekend I stayed with her from Saturday morning to Sunday noon, giving the son a break. She now sleeps in a room that has in it a used hospital bed, two chests for her clothes and a potty chair. There isn't much point to the chair anymore because she is in diapers now and doesn't think about using the chair or going to an actual bathroom. Having the chests in there is new and more convenient. We don't have to worry anymore about her taking the clothes out or storing excrement in the drawers. I bought the bed for her at the Alabama Thrift Store in the summer of 1996. It isn't fully operative—a lot of the wiring is shot—so I guess it wasn't really a bargain, but it does have side railings. We attach restraints to these at night. I noticed last weekend that she has a tendency to draw her legs up and try to throw them out of the bed in between the bars on the left side. If the rails weren't there, she might be partially out of bed.

Yesterday, I brought her home in my pickup as usual. I buckled the seat belt, naturally, but this time she was leaning over toward her door and trying to stick her feet up into the dashboard. This wasn't too distracting until she started to try to stick a foot into the tape deck/radio. Not desirable. I noticed much the same thing today, driving my son's car (Formerly his grandfather's 1984 or 1985 Oldsmobile. It had maybe 34,000 miles on it when we brought it over in 1993.) because he was borrowing my truck to haul some stuff. Again, she was assuming much the same posture, except that she was sprawling back on the seat, her face in a kind of rictus. I don't know if she was in pain or what.

The woman at daycare said that although Mom was eating well, she thought they were going to have to go to puree, which is pretty much what I decided over the weekend. As an addition to her nutritive liquid drink, I had mashed up some canned macaroni and cheese. She was spitting out small shreds of pasta, which caused me to see the futility of it.

WEDNESDAY

Wed, 29 January 97

Monday afternoon, the daycare facility notified my son that they thought Mom needed to be taken to the emergency room. Not too surprising, because her health has definitely worsened over the last week. She has been bleeding a good bit from the rectum, withdrawing further, and has begun to refuse to eat and drink.

My daughter was staying with her this past weekend, and when I went down to my son's house this past Sunday morning, although Mom was still wearing her diaper, she was lying in a dreadful mess—blood, some fecal matter, and urine. My daughter was alarmed and had just tried to telephone me to ask how much blood was a lot of blood.

We washed her up a little and then carried her to the bathroom to do a more thorough cleaning-up. My son had told me that this was what he had been having to do nearly every morning—pick her up and carry her in to sit on something in the tub and hose her down with the shower extension.

Anyway, after she had been cleaned and dressed, we brought her into the dining area to eat. She refused to drink the Equate. What little went in, she swished around in her mouth and eventually spit out. My daughter gave her some of the anti-agitation medicine and her heart medicine, both of which are liquid and given via droppers. Most of that, she seemed to swallow, but she spit out saliva for about 45 minutes thereafter.

On Monday afternoon, when I collected her in response to the call from the daycare facility, it was obvious that she was much worse. She was panting—laboring for breath—with her eyes closed, fairly unresponsive to outside stimuli. At the hospital, they discovered that she was badly dehydrated, bleeding, and had a systemic infection of some sort.

Yesterday morning, when I got off the elevator I could hear the sound of my mother's breathing all the way down the hall. It was rasping—labored—awful.

Although I had missed our doctor on her morning rounds, I was able to talk to her at her office. She says Mom is dying and that she won't be leaving the hospital this time. It could be a matter of only a day or two or maybe a little longer, but she is not going to get better this time. She said there were so many things gone wrong now, probably as a result of her long term refusal to eat or drink enough and also, from simple breakdown of the system, that it wasn't possible to do much of anything now, except try to keep her comfortable.

Also she pointed out that while it might be possible to operate to locate the cause of the bleeding, in the shape my mom's in now, she couldn't reasonably be expected to survive surgery. Mom seems to be comatose—definitely unresponsive to voices. We agreed that a feeding tube should not be used.

I was saved the unpleasantness of breaking the news to my uncle, her brother. While I was gone from the hospital, he got a nurse to level with him about his sister's chances, and by the time I talked to him, he seem relatively resigned. Our doctor, in commenting on the sudden downward turn, remarked that she had seen this kind of thing in a lot of patients. At some point, it seems as if the body or person decides to shut down. It stops eating and drinking and just retreats, achieving the same state as the mind at last.

My mother has lost so much weight that the clothes she used to wear are many sizes too large for her. I had bought her a lot of very attractive, expensive clothes in the first year after she moved to Alabama, but by the summer of 1995, she had already lost so much weight and been so overcome by Alzheimer's that I gave them all to my son's girl friend, who is also petite, to dispose of as she saw fit.

All she has been wearing the last couple of years has been sweat suits and those warm-up outfits. Therefore, I went to the local thrift store yesterday and purchased a couple of dresses, although I don't know whether either of them will fit. We'll see. Although my daughter and I picked out the coffin for my father when he died in 1986, this will be the first funeral for which I will have to make the decisions. It feels very strange. I have called all the closest relatives to alert them—well, I just remembered one I haven't—no, two. I think I'd better wait on that until after the funeral. Otherwise, they might think I expected them to come all the way from Houston. And I don't.

It's odd. After all the negative emotions I have felt toward my mother, the rage, the unevenness—and I still feel so guilty about not doing any better than I have—after all that, I still apparently am going to regret her passing. I suppose this is because it is the end of a unit that consisted of my paternal grandmother, my father, my mother, and me. I am going to be all that's left.

Well, it's time that one moved on. I need to grasp the fact that my life is about me.

GOODBYES

Wed, 29 January 97

I got to the hospital fairly early this morning. One could see no change in my mother. However, I did see the doctor. She said that her estimate was 24 to 48 hours. The lungs are beginning to accumulate fluid, and the heart can't cope. Mom is still comatose.

I just returned from going to the hospital again. Surprisingly enough, my daughter was there sitting with her grandmother. I stayed a little while, but left her to have whatever time she wanted. She remarked that she didn't get to see her grandfather for one last time before he died, which is true. She had been working at a summer theatre in Ogden, Utah, for most of the summer of 1986, but had returned home by then. It had been recognized that my father was in his last days by then and might die at any time. She stayed in Montevallo for her birthday, which was on August 13, but she came over to Water Valley on the 14th. She got there late in the afternoon but didn't go down to the hospital that day. Unfortunately, he died around one A.M. on the morning of the 15th before she saw him.

My older son came over from Georgia today to have a last look at his grandmother. Apparently, he stayed at the hospital for a longish time. One tends to forget that he lived with his grandparents for part of the time when he was going to college at Ole Miss, developing stronger relationships than would otherwise have existed. Probably, there is more emotion involved there than one has realized.

My younger son and I tended to a number of chores today—contacting the respective funeral homes, here and in Water Valley, discussing funding, getting the clothes together, and some other stuff.

As to myself, I thought of one thing that is troubling—this is going to be the end of any chance to mend fences, to make things better, or to ever reach understandings. Of course, that opportunity was gone long ago with my mother's mind, but this is the final irrevocable point in life where all chance slips away.

CATCH-UP

Sat, 01 February 97

Well, after having the doctor tell me on the 29th that Mom had 24–48 hours to live, it is with the usual irony that I report that she is still ticking. In wretched condition, of course, but still hanging in. She seemed to be feeling some pain, so the doctor has prescribed morphine. I don't know how long this will continue.

I'm really dreading the funeral because whereas I am very easy to please, others are more picky. However, it is one more thing to get through, and we will.

SUNDAY

Sun, 02, February 97

As the period of my mother's illness has gone on, I have become more and more aware of how this issue touches so many people. I knew the day was going to come when my mother was dependent on me, but she was always so healthy that my main dread was the one about having her around, taking over my life, as she was wont to do. What happened, though, was that the mind went away, leaving her body to wind down, very slowly. I think this matter of the health care of the elderly is definitely a discussible issue, as much as welfare, taxes, health care and all the rest of it is.

There was a man who had Alzheimer's at the daycare establishment my mother attended, who was in his mid-fifties at most, younger than I. If you don't know it already, Alzheimer's is an awful, awful thing. I never knew. Perhaps no one knows until they experience the effects. But it is out there.

The doctor has prescribed round-the-clock—every four hours—administration of morphine for my mother because something seems to be hurting her. Inasmuch as she has been bleeding constantly and, sometimes profusely, from the rectum for at least two weeks now, the possibility of some painful cause seems quite likely.

My uncle's daughter, who is the same age as my children, has been staying all night with the mom. She flew in from California a day or two ago. This seems to be a vigil that she and her parents—especially her mother, who is a retired Red Cross nurse—seems to want to keep. I suppose it seems insensitive of me, but I see no point in my staying all the time. The nurses are very good to Mom. I don't feel that staying will make me or her feel better. Maybe the anti-depressants have wiped me clean of emotion? I do think that the last four years have wrung me out emotionally to a large extent. I feel as blank as a newly washed slate.

MONDAY

Mon, 03 February 97

I went to the hospital earlier this morning, so as to catch my mother's doctor on her rounds. She said that she had done some thinking yesterday and had decided that, with our permission, she was going to give orders to remove the IV drip. They would leave the entry into the vein so as to be able to administer medication and the morphine to keep her comfortable, but there would be no more fluid administered.

We agreed it was the only reasonable thing to do, given her condition and the impossibility of restoring her to health in mind and body. She continues to bleed, thereby slowly diminishing her blood supply.

It's dreadful, but it seems the only thing to be done.

TUESDAY

Tue, 04 February, 97

I went to the hospital this morning. My cousin had to return to her family in California today. Apparently, she had intended to stay through my mother's death, but not the funeral, which I can certainly understand. My mother had stood by her during the difficult period of her marriage to a Chinese/American. I was proud of the mom for that. Deep down, I love the mom, as so many people do their parents, but I really don't like her very much. I never have that I can remember. We are too different to have ever bonded very well.

Without the IV fluid, my mother is still surviving. The doctor said that as functions slow down, it takes longer. So who knows how long it will take? Some technician came in this morning before I got there, measured her oxygen level, and said that if it drops below a certain point, he will administer oxygen. We told the doctor, and she said that she would leave orders that it not be done. However, one never knows what the nursing staff will do. I'll be going back soon, so I guess we will find out what happened.

My mother has had such an incredibly strong body. One wonders how long she might have lived if she hadn't lost her mind.

THURSDAY

Thu, 06 February 97

I tried two times yesterday to enter the following information here and thought I had succeeded, but for some reason it didn't post. Anyway, I will try again. The string needs closure.

I spent Tuesday afternoon with my mother at the hospital. Many times it looked as if she were about to die, but by the end of the afternoon, the morphine was wearing off, and her lungs weren't clogging as badly. My aunt arrived around 5:00 P.M., and I went home. However, later, at approximately 10:40 P.M., she did die.

It is finally over.

Finis.

CONCLUSION:
Here and Now

SUMMATION

Shortly before my mother's death, I transferred my posts from the message boards of one section of America Online to the message boards of the American Civil Liberties Union, where I had come to know a number of people who contributed posts. I also posted there the information about the last days and her death, which occurred on Tuesday, February 4.

We had made arrangements to have her funeral and burial in Water Valley, Mississippi. With that end in mind, I went to Mississippi on Thursday, February 6. This gave me plenty of time to confer with the officials at the funeral home in Water Valley, see my relatives who live there, and have the standard visitation on the evening of the 7th. My uncle and aunt arrived in time for the visitation at the funeral home on the 7th, as did my daughter and her father, who stayed at the same motel as I. My uncle and aunt stayed at my cousin's house.

My sons, accompanied, respectively, by girl friend and wife, arrived for the funeral on the 8th and returned to Alabama and Georgia that same afternoon after the funeral, as did my uncle and aunt and my daughter and her father. I stayed overnight so as to get a fresh start on Sunday. I've gotten old enough now, that I don't like long end-of-the-day trips, unless they are absolutely necessary.

THANKS I

When I got back home and got around to going online, I was quite surprised to find several messages of condolence had been added to the folder. One of the ACLU hosts spoke of the difficulty of bearing such an irrevocable change in one's life. In response I wrote:

Actually, I would be a fraud if I pretended to be wallowing in grief. My mother has been gone a long time already, leaving behind a shell to be tended. People keep saying that it will hit me after a while. I think the loss of the first parent is the hardest, in my experience, because until then, although one knows it will happen eventually, it has not been imminent. Also, the circumstances make a difference.

I feel right now as if a tremendous burden had been rolled off my back. In the words of Ayn Rand, I—Atlas—have shrugged. I feel light as a feather and as if possibilities were infinite, as, indeed they may be.

THANKS II

Mon, 10 February 97

Another long-time poster expressed gratitude for my having shared the experience with others and playfully speculated on whether my mother might have, as a last gesture, caused the current on-line system screw-ups:

Regarding my mom's ability to mess up the system, it wouldn't have surprised me, but it's funny how people's perceptions differ. So many people back in Water Valley were telling me how sweet my mother was. Of course, sweet, nice, cute, and interesting, etc., are all words that may be interpreted in many, many ways. From my viewpoint my mother was a woman who would expend her last bit of energy to carry out whatever project in which she was engaged.

She did, indeed, put in a lot of time making brownies, cooking green beans, and making pimento cheese spread to give to people at various times. Perhaps some of that has to do with the perceived sweetness, but from my viewpoint a lot of that also had to do with pride and public recognition of her charity. That sounds unkind, I guess, but I mean it as simple realism. She was sometimes very considerate of others, but she could also be incredibly tactless and a professional martyr.

THANKS III

Mon, 10 February 97

Another person said that she had a friend who was experiencing a situation similar to mine and that I had given her the means to express to him that he was not alone in his experience by sending him copies of my posts. She said, further, that I should try to share this with a wider audience. I wrote:

Thank you. As I have said before, although I don't know whether people believe me or not, I hoped, when I set out, that this journalization could be useful to people in some way or another. As life has unfolded since then I have realized over and over what a problem is going to be facing many people. The facilities and possibilities for dealing with the elderly and ill in our country are severely limited.

I can remember how my mother and I fretted over the kind of care my father was receiving during his last few months in the nursing home that was attached to the local hospital. In fact, those circumstances probably more rapidly precipitated his death, although there was no reason at all to wish him to linger by then. He had developed a horrible bedsore and had infected it with fecal matter. What with his disease—Lupus—it became very bad, indeed. Flesh sloughing off down to the bone.

Still, I can now understand how workers in that field might feel. I can deal with blood and bone and flesh, but changing diapers and washing patients would not be things I could do on and on unless my life were dependent on it. In the last weeks of my mother's life, it got where it sometimes seemed I could smell her feces all over the house, in nooks and crannies where she had never been. Probably a peculiarity of my nose because she was not even in my house at that time.

THANKS IV

Mon, 10 February 97

One person sympathized, remarking how his mother frequently inquired of her children as to how they intended to take care of her when the time came. I commented:

Your comment about your mother reminds me of what my mother was always saying when I would visit her.

"What are you going to do?" she would ask. This was a woman who, even when she was thoroughly lost in Alzheimer's, could still run up the hill from her house to the town above and could hoe, squatting like a Russian folk dancer, with one leg extended, so as to get closer to the object of her intent to destroy. It was a little difficult to envision her ever becoming weak. Indeed, it took a long time to wear her body down. Seemingly, at least, a very long time.

My younger son has a friend whom he employed in his heating and cooling business—Marathon Cooling and Heating—who had a maternal grandmother who attended the first daycare center my mom went to. Although he had finished college, he was mostly working odd jobs for the time being while he waited for a promised position to come into being, and so he got to pick up his grandmother from the center.

I remember that his family was really looking forward to Granny going to live with her son for a while. She had lived there before, and it was past time to rotate back. Supposedly, the son's family was getting ready to receive her again, but at the last minute they reneged for some reason. The daughter's family was extremely disappointed, which I can certainly understand, and, so far as I know, they're still having to keep her. I sympathize.

FUNEREAL MATTERS

Mon, 10 February 97

I have been very touched by the messages that you people have left in this folder. Life has seemed so solitary during the last nearly four years that it has been easy to forget that there was a caring world outside the tight circle of the mom, me, my son, his girl friend, my daughter, and my uncle and aunt. I thank you all—those who have posted and those who have empathized silently.

It has been nearly two weeks now—lacking a few hours—since I took my mother to the hospital for her final stay. This last stay was nothing like the hospitalization for her broken hip. She rarely had much degree of consciousness. Truth to tell, she has not been truly lucid in years. There have merely been mechanical responses. During the last couple of days of her life, I could say her name in a brisk manner, much as her mother used to say it, and she would make a noise in response. The doctor, as I have already mentioned, prescribed morphine, so I don't feel that she suffered greatly, except for the filling up of her lungs at the end.

Although I, along with my daughter, had picked out the casket for my father because my mother was too distraught at the time, I had not been involved with the other details of that funeral. Perhaps I should have been. However, because of that event and occasional attendance at other funerals over the years, at least I had some prior knowledge of the typical arrangement of funerals here in the rural South.

Because my mother had lived nearly all her life in Water Valley and because my father was buried there with a double headstone in a plot for which I have the deed, taking her back to Mississippi seemed the logical choice. Therefore, this matter was going to involve two funeral homes.

My son investigated and found that it was necessary to embalm the body in order to carry it into another state. So the local funeral home picked up the body at the hospital and did the embalming work. I gave her clothes to my son to take to the funeral home. As it turned out, the dress looked very good on her. In my opinion, most of the clothes were unnecessary, but, apparently, the funeral home expects people to want their loved ones to be fully dressed for interment. This is somewhat ridiculous, if you ask me, unless one adheres to ancient Egyptian beliefs. We communicated with the funeral home in Water Valley, as did the funeral home here, and the Water Valley firm sent a hearse over to pick up the body.

The local expense for embalming was $925. It's probably more expensive elsewhere. I told the guy I was going to be cremated. He said that kind of thing could be arranged in advance and quoted me a price of roughly $1300+. I'll go ahead and list the expenses for the stuff in Water Valley:

1. The casket itself, the cheapest acceptable one they had: $3010.

2. Basic professional services of funeral director and staff: $1260

3. Dressing, casketing, and cosmetology. This item was probably not only worth what they charged, but more, because she really looked quite beautiful, although emaciated. We hadn't been at all sure that an open casket service was going to be possible: $50.

4. Services for visitation: $230.

5. Services for funeral: $250.

6. Hearse and driver: $120.

7. Flower van and driver: $50.

8. Cemetery tent and grave equipment: $100.

9. Transportation beyond 50 mi. radius: $264

10. Acknowledgment cards: $30.

11. Memorial register: $15.

Total charges from funeral home: $5,379.

Value of 3 burial policies my mother had that she had been paying on since 1986: $1150.

Total paid in cash to funeral home: $4229

There will be a few additional expenses. I will have to pay for the obituary notice in the *Birmingham News*, although the one in the *Shelby County Reporter* will be free. I will also have to pay about $75 for the engraving on the tombstone. The company will bill me directly and separately for that.

I had to pay the City of Water Valley $200 for opening and closing a grave on a weekend, and there was also the matter of $25 to $30 for the preacher. He earned it, in my opinion. A very nice talk, with humor, based upon all the stories that the older members of the church told him about my father and mother. I decided to go with using the Methodist minister because while I am not a Christian anymore, my parents were fervid supporters of their church, and all their hometown friends and relations are Christians. It was my feeling that, except for my uncle who had a very personal stake, it was most important to bring a kind of closure for the community in which they had lived. I think it did and am relatively satisfied with the matter.

LIFE BEGINS ANEW

Tue, 11 February 97

My doctor said, week before last, that when it was all over, I was going to feel like sleeping a lot. I thought it unlikely, but I'm beginning to feel that she was right.

I went to see my therapist today, and while I felt very buoyant going into Birmingham, I don't think I truly communicated my feelings to her. My original appointment to see her had been on the 4th, but I had canceled it the day before, which turned out to be a wise decision.

I'm feeling pretty good attitude-wise, but kind of tired physically, which is a little strange, since I haven't really expended all that much physical energy lately. I had time to think about some things, driving into Birmingham. I had already noticed that I felt different—as if a weight had been lifted. I had been singing along with the radio coming home on Sunday, and I find that I'm smiling these days and singing around the house. This is a change.

It's hard to say whether I have had this feeling that I shouldn't be enjoying or entertaining myself, or whether perhaps I was punishing myself. I do understand that I had come to think that there was little point in trying to achieve happiness or any kind of joy. Certainly I felt that I should not anticipate anything with any notion of pleasure because it was not likely to materialize.

EVALUATION

Mon, 24 February 97

Summing up. What may I say that I have not muttered or screamed already? Reading in the books on Alzheimer's, I note the admonition that the caregivers may need some consideration and be given a little free time. Excellent advice, except that "a little free time," while welcome and necessary, doesn't come close to alleviating the suspicion on the part of the caregiver that the ordeal will never end and that the eventual outcome is going to leave such a load of guilt that the caregiver is going to be bogged down with another problem. I think I am turning out to be lucky with this last. Once I have dealt with money matters and some details, barring some new disaster, my life is going to be mine to do with as I wish. More freedom than I have ever had in my life before. It comes as a daily surprise, to discover that each day doesn't come with a cloud hanging over, but, rather, as something to be savored for whatever distinguishes one day from another.

I think I have no advice, although I do know one thing—this country is going to have to make some decisions and arrangements in the very near future to accommodate the massive problem that awaits us as I and those of the generation behind me achieve old age and begin to need care. That it is going to be a massive problem, I have no doubt, and I admonish those who presume to plan for and deal with matters of this magnitude that they had better get to planning with an intensity they have not applied before. This future seems unavoidable, and it is coming at us steadily. It will arrive. How are we going to deal with it?

TIME'S WINGED CHARIOT

Mon, 26 February 97

For years now—maybe all my life, but I'm not going to stop right now to check it—I have had this rather annoying habit of going along, all chirky—head up, tail up—and then, suddenly, had a great illumination. I will mention this illumination to others and, mostly, they are kind and don't say any of the really scathing things they would be perfectly justified in uttering.

Well, it's happened again, but I haven't gotten to the communication stage, so this time, instead of merely exposing myself to the contempt of my immediate circle, I'm going to let thousands enjoy the feeling of knowing that they are superior to me in prescience.

I turned 60 last week, which was no big deal. I've known for a long time now that the years are piling up, and I have been somewhat blessed in that I have not had to suffer some of the things that other people have had to endure. I am appreciative of that. It strikes me that I have not been sufficiently appreciative.

I used to plan to live forever, but the recent experience with my mother's deterioration kind of took the gloss off my expectations for a while. However, although I'm getting better, it struck me this afternoon that perhaps I should start making some alternative plans, in case something unforeseen occurs.

I got to feeling unwell this afternoon—a low-grade temp of 99, which isn't bad, except that I have been doing this off and on since before Christmas. I went out to buy some Tylenol PM to help me make it through the night, and I got to thinking. Thinking about all those bed-ridden people I saw during my mother's hospitalizations. I haven't ever had to be hospitalized. No serious illnesses. Therefore, I have gone along blithely thinking that "one of these days" I was going to have to get serious about my health.

I am reminded of that little bit in the play and movie, *On Golden Pond*, when Chelsea and her mother are chatting about Chelsea's problems in relation to getting along with her father. Chelsea is saying that one of these days they'll work it out. Her mother asks her when this is going to be. Her father is in his eighties and not in good health. When, exactly, is "one of these days" going to be the right time?

I am 60, and I have some health problems. My mother just died at 83+ of Alzheimer's. My father died ten years ago at 75 from complications of Lupus. His father died at about 55 of a stroke. His mother died at 76+ of strokes and resulting ailments. My mother's mother died in her early eighties of heart problems (and probably complications from diabetes). Her father died when she was about eleven, from complications resulting from a gunshot wound.

Well, let's see. I have already outlived both my grandfathers. If I match my father and his mother, I might have roughly 15–16 years to go. If I match my mother and her mother, I might have 23 years yet. As a matter of fact, I had a great-great uncle—Garvin Chastain—who lived to be over 100 years old, but at significant emotional cost to his relatives. He was a Baptist missionary to Mexico long ago and wrote a book about it. Quite a character!

The point is—I am 60. I can probably number my years now. If I am ever going to get in shape or conquer those little habits that might land me in a comatose state in a hospital bed, now is the time to do it. My future depends on what I do right now, and every tomorrow that follows, from now on. I am not afraid to die. I am not afraid to contemplate my end. Still it behooves me to stop living my life like a chicken with its head just wrung off, flopping around as life drains out.

I am not helpless. Once upon a time we had more monetary resources than we do now. I sold things off too hastily and let my emotions guide me rather than my head in the handling of money. But I am not helpless or without abilities.

I am *only* 60. I may have many, many years awaiting me, and I fully believe that I can do any thing I choose to do—but I need to get started doing them!

978-0-595-48139-2
0-595-48139-6

www.ingramcontent.com/pod-product-compliance
Lightning Source LLC
Chambersburg PA
CBHW020335290526
45785CB00005B/2035